BUNIONS SURGERY RECOVERY DIET PLAN

Comprehensive Guide Unlocking The Secrets
of nutrition after Surgery Success, Nourishing
Meal Plans, Recipes And Practical Tips For
Optimal Health And Wellness)

DR. ALLAN FREDA

Contents

Bunion Surgery Recovery Diet Plan" provides a thorough guide to the best post-surgery nutrition for people who have had bunion surgery.

It also offers insightful information about the importance of a well-planned diet in fostering healing and long-term wellness after the surgical procedure.

Within the book, readers can anticipate receiving professional guidance on creating healing recipes, personalized meal plans, and vital advice for maintaining overall health following the procedure.

By emphasizing nutrition and assisting in the healing process, this book acts as a reliable resource for people who have recently been diagnosed, assisting them in achieving a successful and satisfying rehabilitation journey.

Disclaimer

The information in this book is for informational purposes only and should not replace professional medical advice, diagnosis, or treatment. Always consult your physician or a qualified health provider regarding any medical concerns. Do not disregard professional medical advice or delay seeking it based on information in this book.

CHAPTER 1
UNDERSTANDING BUNION SURGERY RECOVERY

Overview of Bunion Surgery

Bunion surgery, also referred to as a bunionectomy, is a procedure used to treat a bunion, which is a painful bony bump that develops on the joint at the base of the big toe.

This condition, also known as hallux valgus, causes the big toe to point toward the second toe, causing misalignment of the joint and leading to pain, inflammation, and difficulty walking. The goal of bunion surgery is to realign the joint, relieve pain, and restore normal function to the affected foot. Depending on the severity of the bunion and the patient's particular needs, different surgical techniques are used, such as osteotomy (cutting and realigning bones), arthrodesis (joint fusion), and ostectomy (removing the bony bump).

Keys to Post-Operative Care

To minimize complications and maximize results, patients should follow the surgeon's post-operative care instructions. These instructions may include keeping the foot elevated to reduce swelling, wearing supportive footwear or a surgical boot to protect the foot, and participating in prescribed exercises to improve mobility and prevent stiffness. Patients are also advised to avoid putting weight on the operated foot for a specified period and to gradually return to normal activities under the guidance of their healthcare provider. After bunion surgery, patients usually go through a period of recovery that involves rest, elevation, and physical therapy to promote healing and restore strength and flexibility to the foot.

The Role of Nutrition in Healing

Poor nutrition can hinder the body's ability to heal effectively, prolong recovery time, and increase the risk of post-operative complications. Therefore, paying attention to dietary intake during the recovery period is essential.

Following bunion surgery, nutrition plays a crucial role in the healing process. A well-balanced diet rich in essential nutrients supports the body's healing mechanisms, strengthens the immune system, and promotes tissue repair. Adequate protein intake is particularly important for tissue regeneration and muscle recovery. Vitamins and minerals like vitamin C, vitamin D, calcium, and zinc are essential for bone health and immune function. Additionally, maintaining hydration is crucial for proper wound healing and preventing complications like infection.

Suggestions for an Effective Rehabilitation Process

In order to facilitate healing and maintain long-term well-being, developing a thorough recovery plan after bunion surgery requires not only adhering to medical guidance and physical therapy but also implementing a nutrient-dense diet.

The following tips can help you create a successful recovery journey:

1. Speak with a healthcare professional: To make sure that your nutritional needs are satisfied during the recovery period, speak with your healthcare provider or a registered dietitian before making any dietary changes. They can offer individualized recommendations based on your medical history, surgical procedure, and personal preferences.

2. Emphasize whole meals high in critical nutrients: Fruits, vegetables, lean meats, whole grains, and healthy fats are just a few examples of foods high in nutrients that offer the vitamins, minerals, antioxidants, and phytonutrients required for healing and sustaining general health.

3. Make protein consumption a priority. To promote tissue repair, muscle recovery, and immunological function, include enough of

protein sources in your diet, such as poultry, fish, eggs, dairy products, legumes, nuts, and seeds.

Aim for a balanced intake of protein throughout the day to improve healing.

4. Remain hydrated: To help good wound healing, drink lots of fluids, such as water, herbal teas, and electrolyte-rich drinks. Adequate hydration is crucial for the transportation of nutrients, the removal of toxins, and the maintenance of general health.

5. Eat foods with anti-inflammatory qualities: To lessen inflammation and encourage healing, include foods like fatty fish (salmon, mackerel, and sardines), olive oil, nuts, seeds, berries, leafy greens, and turmeric in your diet.

6. Steer clear of inflammatory foods: Reduce your intake of processed meals, sugary snacks, refined carbs, trans fats, and excessive alcohol, since these can worsen inflammation, weaken your immune system, and impede your body's ability to heal.

7. Watch portion sizes: Eating balanced meals and snacks at regular intervals will help control blood sugar levels and give sustained energy throughout the day. This will help prevent overeating and promote weight management throughout the recovery phase.

8. Listen to your body: Keep an eye out for any food allergies or digestive problems that may surface throughout the healing process, and make the appropriate dietary adjustments to support comfort and well-being. Pay attention to how your body reacts to various meals.

Along with supporting optimal healing, improving physical function, and enhancing overall health and wellness over time, adhering to these guidelines and incorporating a well-balanced diet into your bunion surgery recovery plan can also help you work closely with healthcare providers and get valuable guidance and support from a registered dietitian during your recovery process.

CHAPTER 2

BUILDING A FOUNDATION: ESSENTIAL NUTRIENTS FOR HEALING

Following bunion surgery, a structured recovery diet plan is necessary to promote healing and guarantee the best possible results. This extensive guide explores the significance of key nutrients, offering high-protein recipes for bone health, vitamin-rich dishes for immune system support, and mineral-rich meals for tissue repair.

Summary of Vital Nutrients:

Understanding the importance of vital nutrients is crucial for a successful healing process in the aftermath of bunion surgery. These nutrients are important for many physiological functions, such as immune function, bone remodeling, and tissue repair. Proteins are the building blocks of tissue regeneration and repair, helping to synthesize collagen and elastin, which are vital components of connective tissue.

Vitamins, like vitamin C, support the immune system, promoting wound healing and lowering the risk of infection. Minerals, such as calcium and magnesium, are vital for bone health, supporting the formation and strength of bones and assisting in the healing process post-surgery.

Recipes Packed with Protein for Tissue Repair:

Proteins are critical for muscle recovery and tissue repair after bunion surgery. Including protein-rich recipes in the post-surgery diet can help to maximize healing and recovery. Lean protein sources, like fish, poultry, legumes, and tofu, should be a mainstay of meals. Main courses such as baked salmon or grilled chicken breast seasoned with herbs and spices are filling and nutritious. Vegetarians and vegans can get their fill of protein and vital vitamins and minerals from lentil stew or chickpea curry.

Snacks like Greek yogurt with nuts or hummus with whole-grain crackers are easy ways to increase protein intake during the day. Protein-rich ingredients, like whey protein powder, almond milk, and fruits, can

Vitamin-Heavy Recipes to Boost Immunity:

A robust immune system is essential for combating infections and promoting wound healing post-bunion surgery. Incorporating vitamin-rich dishes into the recovery diet can bolster immune function and support overall wellness.

Citrus fruits, berries, and leafy greens are excellent sources of vitamin C, a potent antioxidant that aids in collagen synthesis and immune modulation. Adding oranges, strawberries, and spinach to salads or smoothies can provide a refreshing burst of vitamins and minerals. Vitamin

E-rich foods, such as nuts, seeds, and avocado, possess anti-inflammatory properties and promote tissue repair. Including a variety of colorful fruits and vegetables in meals ensures a diverse array of vitamins and antioxidants, enhancing immune function and promoting optimal recovery. Additionally, incorporating immune-boosting herbs and spices, such as ginger, garlic, and turmeric, into recipes can further enhance the therapeutic benefits of the post-surgery diet. By prioritizing vitamin-rich foods, individuals can fortify their immune defenses and support the healing process following bunion surgery.

Mineral-Rich Meals to Support Bone Health:

Maintaining bone health is paramount for individuals recovering from bunion surgery, as adequate mineral intake supports bone remodeling and fracture healing. Incorporating mineral-infused meals into the post-surgery diet can fortify bones and expedite recovery. Calcium-rich foods, such as dairy products, leafy greens, and fortified plant-based milk, should be consumed regularly to support bone density and strength. Incorporating yogurt parfaits with granola and fresh fruit or spinach and cheese omelets into breakfast routines can provide a calcium-rich start to the day. Magnesium, another essential mineral for bone health, can be found in nuts, seeds, whole grains, and leafy greens. Incorporating magnesium-rich foods into meals, such as quinoa salad with almonds and vegetables or pumpkin seed-crusted tofu, can enhance bone metabolism and support the healing process.

Additionally, vitamin D, obtained through sunlight exposure and dietary sources like fatty fish and fortified foods, is crucial for calcium absorption and bone mineralization. Ensuring adequate intake of these essential minerals supports bone health and facilitates optimal recovery following bunion surgery.

CHAPTER 3

CREATING HEALING MEALS: RECIPES FOR EACH STAGE OF RECOVERY

Following bunion surgery, it's critical to focus on diet in order to optimize the healing process.

A thoughtful post-surgery diet plan can help reduce inflammation, encourage tissue repair, and accelerate overall recovery. This detailed guide walks you through the different stages of recovery and guides creating healing meals, complete with recipes specific to each stage.

Light and Comforting Foods during the First Few Days

Your feet may be swollen, tender, and sensitive in the early days after bunion surgery, so it's important to concentrate on eating soft, gentle, easy-to-chew foods. Choose foods low in sodium to avoid water retention and inflammation.

Include lots of fruits and vegetables to support healing with vitamins, minerals, and antioxidants; smoothies made with leafy greens, berries, and protein-rich ingredients like yogurt or tofu can be a great option for a nutrient-dense, easily-absorbed meal; soups and broths made from bone broth or vegetable stock can provide hydration and necessary nutrients without putting undue strain on your digestive tract.

Moving Towards More Textural Cuisine

You can gradually add more textured foods to your diet as the swelling goes down. To support muscle repair and recovery, try including lean proteins like chicken, fish, tofu, or legumes. Whole grains like quinoa, brown rice, or oatmeal can provide sustained energy and important nutrients like fiber and B vitamins. Adding a variety of colorful fruits and vegetables can help provide a range of vitamins, minerals, and antioxidants to support overall health and healing. Try roasting or steaming vegetables, salads, and stir-fries to add variety and flavor to your meals while still prioritizing ease of chewing and digestion.

Making the Switch to Regular Eating Routines

After bunion surgery, you can gradually return to your regular eating habits. The key is to incorporate a balanced diet that consists of a variety of whole foods from all food groups. Try to eat half your plate with fruits and vegetables, a quarter with lean proteins, and a quarter with whole grains.

You can also incorporate healthy fats from sources like avocado, nuts, seeds, and olive oil to provide essential fatty acids to support inflammation and promote healing. To avoid overeating or discomfort, pay attention to your body's hunger and fullness cues. Finally, stay hydrated by drinking lots of water throughout the day and avoiding sugary and alcoholic beverages.

Tasty and Nutritious Recipes for Prolonged Wellness

Following bunion surgery, it is crucial to continue putting long-term wellness first. Try delicious and nourishing recipes that use a range of whole foods and herbs and spices to add flavor without adding too many calories or sodium.

You can also support inflammation and promote overall health by including antioxidant-rich ingredients like turmeric, ginger, garlic, and citrus fruits in your meals. You can also keep meals interesting and flavorful by experimenting with different cooking techniques like grilling, baking, steaming, and sautéing. Finally, pay attention to your body's signals and adjust your diet as necessary to support continued healing and long-term wellness.

To sum up, creating a healing diet plan following bunion surgery entails starting with soft and gentle foods, working your way up to more textured fare as healing progresses, returning to regular eating schedules, and incorporating flavorful and nourishing recipes for long-term wellness. You can also support optimal healing and recovery by emphasizing nutrient-dense foods, staying hydrated, and paying attention to your body's cues.

CHAPTER 4
EASY MEAL PLANNING: SUCCESS STRATEGIES

Meal planning is a crucial part of a successful diet plan for recovering from bunion surgery. It entails carefully organizing and preparing meals so that the body gets the nutrients it needs for healing and general wellness. By putting these strategies into practice, people who are having bunion surgery can maximize their recovery and support long-term health goals. This in-depth guide covers all the different facets of meal planning, such as batch cooking and meal prep, creating balanced and varied menus, tailoring recipes to specific dietary needs, and implementing time-saving strategies for busy schedules.

Advice for Batch Cooking and Meal Preparation:

Meal prep and batch cooking are invaluable strategies for individuals recovering from bunion surgery as they streamline the process of meal preparation and ensure access to healthy, nourishing meals throughout the recovery period. To effectively incorporate meal prep and batch cooking into the recovery diet plan, it is essential to set aside dedicated time each week for planning and execution.

 Start by selecting recipes that are suitable for batch cooking and can be easily portioned and stored for later consumption. These may include soups, stews, casseroles, and grain-based dishes such as quinoa or brown rice. Invest in quality storage containers to keep prepared meals fresh and organized in the refrigerator or freezer.

Additionally, consider investing in kitchen appliances such as a slow cooker or Instant Pot to simplify the cooking process and minimize hands-on time. By dedicating a few hours each week to meal prep and batch cooking, individuals can ensure access to nutritious meals without the stress of daily cooking.

Making Varied and Balanced Menus:

A key aspect of a successful bunion surgery recovery diet plan is creating balanced and varied menus that provide a wide range of nutrients necessary for healing and overall well-being. When planning meals, aim to incorporate a diverse selection of fruits, vegetables, whole grains, lean proteins, and healthy fats to ensure comprehensive nutrition.

Focus on incorporating foods rich in vitamins, minerals, and antioxidants known for their anti-inflammatory and immune-boosting properties, such as leafy greens, berries, nuts, seeds, and fatty fish like salmon or trout. Experiment with different cooking methods and flavor profiles to keep meals interesting and enjoyable. For example, try roasting vegetables with herbs and spices, adding fresh herbs and citrus zest to salads, or marinating proteins in homemade sauces or marinades. Additionally, consider incorporating plant-based meals such as vegetarian or vegan options to increase fiber intake and support digestive health. By prioritizing variety and balance in meal planning, individuals can optimize their nutrient intake and support the body's recovery process.

Adapting Recipes to Specific Dietary Requirements:

Another crucial aspect of meal planning for bunion surgery recovery is adjusting recipes to accommodate individual dietary needs and preferences. Whether following specific dietary restrictions or preferences, such as gluten-free, dairy-free, or vegetarian/vegan diets, it is essential to tailor recipes accordingly to ensure both nutritional adequacy and enjoyment of meals. Start by familiarizing yourself with alternative ingredients and substitutes that align with dietary preferences or restrictions. For example, use gluten-free flour blends in baking recipes, swap dairy milk for plant-based alternatives like almond or oat milk, or substitute tofu or legumes for meat in protein-based dishes. Experiment with different flavor combinations and cooking techniques to create satisfying meals that meet individual dietary needs without compromising taste or nutrition. Additionally, consider consulting with a registered dietitian or nutritionist for personalized guidance and support in navigating dietary modifications during the recovery period. By adapting recipes to individual dietary needs, individuals can maintain a nourishing and enjoyable diet that supports their recovery and long-term health goals.

Including Time-Saving Strategies for Demanding Schedules:

For individuals with busy schedules, incorporating time-saving techniques into meal planning can be instrumental in maintaining a healthy and balanced diet during the bunion surgery recovery process. One effective strategy is to prioritize simple and efficient meal options that require minimal preparation and cooking time.

This may include quick and easy recipes such as salads, wraps, stir-fries, or grain bowls that can be assembled with minimal effort.

Additionally, consider utilizing convenience foods such as pre-cut vegetables, canned beans, and precooked grains or proteins to streamline meal preparation further. Another time-saving technique is to make use of leftovers by repurposing them into new meals or incorporating them into future recipes.

For example, leftover roasted vegetables can be added to salads or grain bowls, while cooked grains or proteins can be used as a base for soups or stir-fries. By implementing time-saving techniques and prioritizing efficiency in meal planning, individuals can overcome barriers to healthy eating and maintain a nourishing diet despite a busy schedule.

Ultimately, meal planning is a crucial part of recovering from bunion surgery because it guarantees access to nourishing meals that promote healing and long-term wellness. By implementing the above-mentioned strategies, people can optimize nutrition and support overall health and well-being, simplify the meal preparation process, design varied and balanced menus, cater to specific dietary requirements, and incorporate time-saving strategies for busy schedules.

CHAPTER 5
MINDFUL EATING FOR SUITABLE HEALTH

Using a mindful eating strategy can make a big difference in the speed at which healing from bunion surgery proceeds as well as overall wellbeing. Mindful eating entails being fully present and mindful of the eating experience, from the taste and texture of food to the bodily sensations it evokes. This holistic approach to nourishment not only supports physical healing but also fosters emotional well-being, which speeds up healing and promotes long-term health.

The Value of Intentional Eating in the Healing Process

Because mindful eating can improve the body's healing processes, it is especially important during the healing phase after bunion surgery. After surgery, the body needs enough nutrition to support tissue repair, lower inflammation, and increase immunity.

Mindful eating makes sure that every meal contains the vital vitamins, minerals, and antioxidants needed for optimal healing. It also helps people avoid overeating, which can impede recovery by putting undue strain on the digestive system.

Additionally, by chewing food slowly and thoroughly, the body can break down nutrients more efficiently, supporting the rebuilding of tissues damaged during surgery. Mindful eating also encourages people to choose nutrient-dense foods that provide energy to the body and support cellular regeneration, which is necessary for repairing the affected area. All of these benefits maximize the benefits of the post-surgery diet plan.

Methods for Appreciating Every Bite

To fully savor and appreciate each bite, mindful eating involves using a variety of techniques. One such technique is to use all of the senses during the eating process. This involves observing the colors, textures, and aromas of the food before taking a bite to enhance the sensory experience. It also involves chewing to heighten awareness and satisfaction by focusing on the taste and mouthfeel of each bite.

Eating slowly and mindfully is another way to enjoy every bite of food. People can fully experience the flavors and textures of their meals by taking their time to chew and pausing between bites.

This methodical approach not only improves the pleasure of eating but also facilitates better digestion and nutrient absorption. Moreover, by observing how different foods make one feel, people can make more informed dietary decisions that will support overall wellness and vitality during the healing process.

For those having bunion surgery, food becomes more than just sustenance during the healing phase.

Taking this approach can help patients develop a healthy relationship with food, supporting both physical and emotional healing. By selecting nutrient-dense foods that aid in the body's healing process, patients can actively participate in their recovery while savoring tasty and fulfilling meals.

Comfort foods, like warm soups, stews, and herbal teas, can soothe the body and mind, relieving discomfort and promoting relaxation. Additionally, sharing meals with loved ones can create a sense of connection and support, enhancing the healing journey and promoting overall well-being. All of these benefits can be achieved by including comfort foods in the post-surgery diet plan.

Gratitude Practices for Nutrition and Well-Being

To cultivate a deeper appreciation for the healing properties of meals, people can cultivate a gratitude practice that can improve the mindful eating experience and support overall wellbeing during the recovery process. This shift in perspective not only creates a positive relationship with food, but it also fosters feelings of abundance and contentment.

In addition, cultivating gratitude for the body's healing and recovery capacity can help people feel resilient and empowered. By recognizing the body's inherent wisdom and healing capacity, people can approach the healing process with hope and assurance. Gratitude for the assistance of medical professionals, family members, and caregivers can also help people feel connected to a community and offer extra emotional support during trying times.

In summary, mindful eating is essential to promoting optimal healing during the recuperation phase following bunion surgery. By adopting mindful eating practices, like appreciating every bite, accepting food as a source of comfort and healing, and cultivating gratitude for sustenance and wellness, people can improve their healing process and long-term wellness. They can also prioritize foods high in nutrients, use their senses during eating, and adopt a positive outlook to maximize their post-surgery diet plan for overall health and optimal healing.

CHAPTER 6

INTEGRATIVE APPROACHES TO HEALING: BEYOND THE PLATE

Beyond the operating room, bunion surgery recovery is a complex process. Surgical intervention corrects the structural problems, but appropriate post-operative care—including diet—is critical to healing and reducing pain.

To achieve optimal recovery, you must take a holistic approach that includes not only dietary considerations but also gentle movement and exercise, stress management techniques, improving sleep quality, and creating a supportive environment.

We go into great detail about each of these aspects in this comprehensive guide to help you on your path to long-term wellness following bunion surgery.

Exercise and movement should be gradually resumed after bunion surgery to strengthen muscles, increase circulation, and improve range of motion. Before beginning any exercise program, it is important to speak with your healthcare provider to make sure it is appropriate for your recovery period and your particular surgical needs.

Early in the healing process, low-impact exercises like swimming, walking, or stationary cycling can be helpful because they minimize swelling, prevent stiffness, and improve joint mobility without putting undue strain on the surgical site.

Short sessions should be started and the duration and intensity should be increased gradually as tolerated.

It can also be beneficial to include stretches that target the feet, ankles, and lower legs. Caution should be used when performing toe curls, ankle circles, and calf stretches to minimize soreness and facilitate recovery.

It's critical to pay attention to your body and refrain from overdoing it or engaging in painful or uncomfortable activities. Your physical therapist or doctor may offer tailored advice on appropriate exercises and adjustments depending on your specific recovery trajectory.

Techniques for Stress Management in Healing:

Stress may worsen pain, slow down healing, and impair general health, so it's critical to manage it throughout the healing phase after bunion surgery. Using stress-reduction strategies in your daily routine helps ease tension and encourage serenity and relaxation.

Devote some time each day to practicing mindfulness techniques, even if it's just for a short while, to reap the advantages of lower stress levels and increased mental clarity.

These techniques include progressive muscle relaxation, deep breathing exercises, and meditation.

Reducing stress may also be accomplished by keeping an optimistic mindset and concentrating on the advancements you've made. Surround yourself with people who are encouraging and there to help when required.

Moreover, throughout the healing process, taking part in enjoyable and soothing activities like reading, listening to music, or going outside can aid in promoting emotional well-being and serve as a distraction from discomfort.

Improving the Quality of Sleep for the Best Recovery:

After bunion surgery, the body needs good quality sleep to mend and recover because it helps with hormone regulation, tissue regeneration, and energy replenishment. However, pain and altered mobility can interfere with sleep cycles, making it difficult to obtain enough sleep.

Better sleep quality may be achieved by establishing a regular sleep pattern and creating a sleep-friendly atmosphere. To help your body's internal clock function properly, try to go to bed and wake up at the same time every day, especially on weekends.

Investing in supportive mattresses and pillows, reducing light and noise distractions, and elevating your feet slightly with pillows may all assist create a comfortable sleeping environment.

Close to bedtime, steer clear of stimulants like caffeine and gadgets that might keep you from falling asleep. Instead, practice soothing activities like reading or taking a warm bath to let your body know it's time to unwind.

See your healthcare practitioner for advice on pain management techniques or safe sleep aids to utilize throughout the healing process if pain or discomfort does not subside.

Creating a Healing-Supportive Environment:

After bunion surgery, recovery can be both physically and psychologically taxing, so it's important to create a healing and well-being-promoting environment. Surround yourself with people who care about you, your loved ones, and medical professionals who can support and encourage you as you heal.

Openly discuss your recovery objectives, worries, and any help you might need with your support network. Having a solid support system can reduce feelings of loneliness and give comfort when things go hard.

Assign duties and responsibilities as necessary to reduce stress and give yourself enough time to concentrate on your recuperation. Don't be afraid to ask for help when you need it—whether it's with food preparation, housework, or transportation to doctor's appointments.

Apart from the assistance of family and friends, you should also think about adopting assistive devices or adaptive equipment to help with mobility and independence while recovering.

Small adjustments like using a shower chair or walker may make daily activities easier to do and lower the chance of accidents or falls.

Throughout the healing process, don't forget to put self-care first, pay attention to your body's signals, acknowledge any tiny victories, and have patience and compassion for yourself while you work through the difficulties of recovering from bunion surgery.

To sum up, a comprehensive recovery plan should take into account more than just dietary modifications when it comes to bunion surgery.

It should also incorporate stress management techniques, prioritize quality sleep, incorporate gentle movement and exercise, and foster a supportive environment.

By addressing these factors collectively, people can maximize their healing process and promote long-term wellness and mobility.

CHAPTER 7

INDULGENT TREATS AND SPECIAL OCCASION RECIPES: CELEBRATING SUCCESS

The road to recovery from bunion surgery can be difficult, but it's important to recognize and appreciate small victories along the way. Rich desserts, appetizing party fare, and festive feasts can all be incorporated into the recovery diet to help boost spirits and keep a positive outlook. But to promote healing and long-term wellness, moderation in indulgence should be balanced with nutritional knowledge.

Sweet Treats for Festive Occasions

Desserts are a satisfying experience that adds a sweet touch to recuperation following bunion surgery. Sweets such as homemade fruit sorbets, freshly baked cookies, or rich chocolate mousse can offer comfort and gratification during celebratory moments.

Desserts made with healthy ingredients, like whole grains, fresh fruits, and natural sweeteners, can be more nutritious while still satisfying cravings. Dessert recipes that are high in antioxidants, vitamins, and minerals can also benefit the body's healing process and overall health.

Party Foods That Will Please Everyone During Social Events

Events and social gatherings are times to celebrate, but they can also pose difficulties for those recovering from bunion surgery. It is important to plan appetizing party foods that satisfy a large number of palates while simultaneously adhering to dietary needs and preferences.

There are many options available to satisfy a large number of people, ranging from filling appetizers like stuffed mushrooms and vegetable skewers to main courses like grilled salmon with citrus salsa or roasted vegetable quinoa salad.

Adding nutrient-dense ingredients, such as lean proteins, vibrant vegetables, and whole grains, to party dishes not only helps them heal but also supports overall health and vitality.

Joyous Meals for Holidays and Particular Occasions

Holidays and special occasions are occasions to get together with loved ones and celebrate customs and foods. Following bunion surgery, taking part in celebratory feasts may require some modifications to account for dietary needs and restrictions.

Arranging holiday menus with filling dishes like roasted turkey with cranberry quinoa stuffing, roasted root vegetables, and pumpkin soup can promote healing and a sense of coziness while healing from the surgery. Adding seasonal ingredients and spices to celebratory recipes can boost flavor and nutritional value.

A balanced diet plan that supports optimal healing and long-term wellness can be created by consulting with a healthcare professional or registered dietitian. While indulging in celebratory treats and special occasion recipes can be enjoyable, it's important to balance indulgence with nutritional wisdom during bunion surgery recovery. Choosing healthier alternatives to traditional ingredients, such as using whole grains instead of refined flour or substituting sugar for natural sweeteners, can help reduce inflammation and promote healing. Integrating nutrient-dense foods like leafy greens, lean proteins, and healthy fats into the recovery diet can provide essential vitamins and minerals needed for tissue repair and immune function.

Chapter 8

Maintaining Health After Recovery: Extended Dietary Approaches

Creating Lifelong Healthy Eating Habits:

Optimal recovery from bunion surgery necessitates sufficient nutrients to support tissue healing, reduce inflammation, and promote overall well-being. As such, moving from a post-surgery diet to a sustainable, lifelong approach involves embracing whole, nutrient-dense foods while minimizing processed and inflammatory ones.

A bunion surgery recovery diet plan goes beyond the immediate post-operative phase and instead focuses on fostering long-term wellness. At the beginning of this journey, it is critical to establish healthy eating habits.

Including Foods That Are Good for Bunions in Regular Meals:

Including bunion-friendly foods in daily meals is crucial for long-term wellness because they not only aid in the healing process but also enhance overall joint health and mobility. Anti-inflammatory foods like fatty fish high in omega-3 fatty acids, vibrant fruits and vegetables high in antioxidants, and whole grains full of fiber and vital nutrients are important parts of a bunion-friendly diet. You can also minimize tissue damage and lower your risk of complications after surgery by including foods high in collagen, zinc, and vitamins C and E. By making these nutrient-dense foods a priority in daily meal planning, people can maximize their recovery and lower their chance of developing bunions again.

Preserving Moderation and Balance for General Well-Being:

A sustainable approach to eating that supports both physical and mental well-being is fostered by striking a balance between nourishing foods and occasional indulgences.

While it's important to focus on nutrient-dense foods, it's equally important to enjoy a variety of foods in moderation. Incorporating treats or indulgences occasionally can help prevent feelings of deprivation and support long-term adherence to a healthy eating pattern. However, it's important to be mindful of portion sizes and frequency to avoid unduly impeding the progress made during recovery.

Proceeding on the Path to Abundant Health and Joy:

Following a particular diet plan is not the only way to continue the journey to vibrant health and happiness after bunion surgery; it also entails taking a holistic approach to wellness, which includes making regular physical activity a priority, learning how to manage stress, getting enough sleep, and building a supportive social network. These lifestyle choices enhance a diet rich in nutrients and help achieve long-term health outcomes. Additionally, keeping lines of communication open with healthcare providers and seeking regular follow-up care can help address any concerns or challenges that may arise. By adopting a holistic approach to wellness, people can maximize their recovery from bunion surgery and improve their overall quality of life for years to come.

SUMMARY

After bunion surgery, recovery is more than just physical; it's about feeding the body, mind, and soul. In this extensive guide, we have covered everything you need to know about post-surgery nutrition, meal planning, mindful eating, holistic recovery methods, and maintaining wellness after the initial healing phase.

Recognizing the role that nutrition plays in healing, we have examined the essential nutrients required for immune function, bone health, and tissue repair. Every component of the diet, from protein-rich dishes to vitamin-rich recipes and mineral-infused meals, has been carefully designed to maximize healing.

In addition, we have offered a guide for creating therapeutic meals at each phase of recuperation, ranging from tender and mild dishes for the first few days to savory and filling recipes for long-term health. We have also explained meal planning techniques to make the process easier and guarantee a variety of well-balanced menus catered to specific dietary requirements.

A focus on holistic approaches to recovery, such as gentle movement, stress management, and quality sleep, has been placed on mindful eating as a practice that not only promotes optimal healing but also cultivates gratitude, savors each bite, and embraces food as a source of comfort and nourishment.

It's important to strike a balance between enjoyment and nutritional knowledge when we celebrate success with decadent treats and recipes for special occasions. Looking beyond the short-term recovery, we have outlined long-term dietary strategies aimed at sustaining wellness, incorporating bunion-friendly foods into everyday meals, and fostering habits for vibrant health and happiness.

To put it simply, this book is a lifesaver of information and encouragement for people who are struggling to recover from bunion surgery.

By adhering to the ideas presented in these chapters, people can set out on a path that leads to long-term health, healing, and nourishment—thus guaranteeing a more promising and healthier future.

www.ingramcontent.com/pod-product-compliance
Lightning Source LLC
Chambersburg PA
CBHW070824290526
45795CB00002B/837